A PEACEFUL WINTER SKI

A meditative story to massage your body
and relax your mind

The complete
NatureBody® Connection
program is available at

www.aquaterramassage.com

A NATUREBODY® MASSAGE STORY

A Peaceful
WINTER
SKI

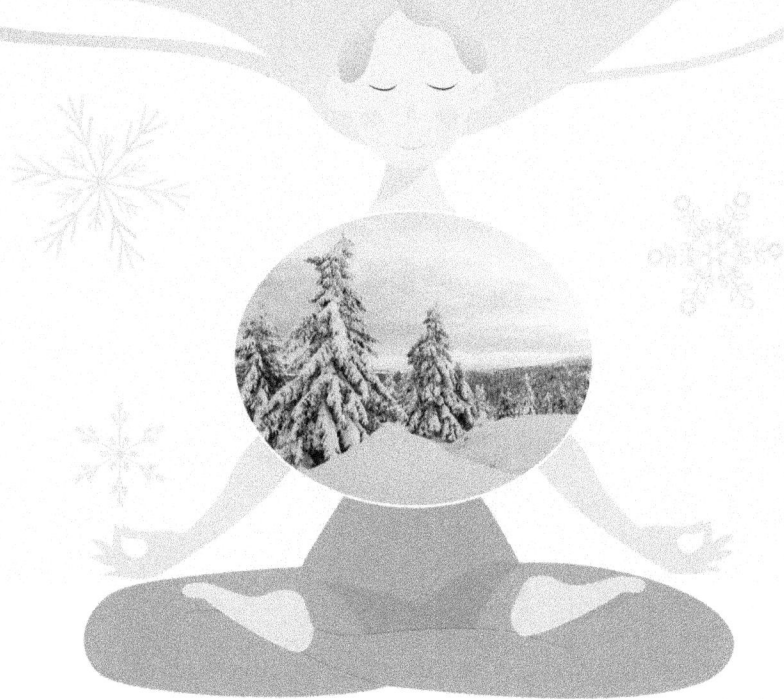

A meditative story to massage your body
and relax your mind

FAYE KRIPPNER *and* ERIK KRIPPNER

Cover art provided by Envato Elements. Cover design by Faye Krippner and Erik Krippner.

Release Date for First Printed Edition 2023.

Media Inquiries: If you would like to contact the authors, please send an email to press@aquaterramassage.com.

Faye Krippner, B.A., LMT and Erik Krippner, B.S., LMT have been licensed by the Oregon Board of Massage Therapy since 2003. Oregon License Numbers: 10233 & 10234

Experience the entire NatureBody® Connection at
www.aquaterramassage.com

Dedicated to your maturing self

as you seek balance

and find wholeness with the seasons.

Index of Reflections

Contents

How to Use This Book

Humans have lived in balance with our bodies and the earth for 2.6 million years. Our bodies are designed for this planet. It is natural to walk on uneven ground, climb mountains, run long distances, swim, and most of all, to deeply breathe fresh air. Our wild planet heals and strengthens us by making us more flexible and fluid.

Your body is born of this earth. Earth is here to support you. Unfortunately, the stresses of life pull us off balance, and can leave us feeling physically sore and mentally anxious. This creative journey into relaxation is a way to remember your natural balance and create new muscle memories.

As massage therapists, we understand how a relaxed body feels: how it breathes, how it moves, how it is balanced in space. This NatureBody® massage story shares the full spectrum of massage: body, mind and spirit. Our intention is to empower you to find healing within yourself.

Visualization can have powerful effects on your body.[1] In this guided visualization, you will exercise your mind and imagination to deeply relax and bring your body back to center.

If you are injured or your ability to move is limited, then visualization is even more important! Studies have shown that when you imagine moving, the same areas of your brain activate as if you are actually moving those specific muscles.[2] Through visualization, you are virtually exercising your body.

We are intending for you to have a tangible, physical response to the ideas in this book. The power of this story lies in the vividness of your imagination. Read slowly. Pause. Use all of your senses to experience the story. Imagine the changes in humidity. Feel the gentle breeze on your skin. Hear the soothing sound of the wind. Smell the fresh scent of the life around you. Use your vibrant imagination to experience every detail in this story.

Put yourself in the story. Try to experience every sensation in your body. If you feel like moving, do it! Trust your instincts. Imagine what it feels like to move through the story: your muscles warming and stretching... your breathing deepening... your heartbeat slowing as you deeply relax. Let these sensations come to you at the speed of thought. This isn't about concentrating as much as it is about experiencing.

Each time you practice visualizing this story, your experience will become more vibrant. Your body is your wilderness to explore and understand. Your mind is your canvas for new muscle memories.

The Reflections are our personal notes to you. They offer you insight into some of the concepts in the story. Use them to spark your own creative thoughts about connection and healing.

The Notes section is full of wonderful articles and books that we have selected for you. If you feel interested in a topic, we highly recommend you look at the notes to explore the topic further.

The Journal at the end of the book gives you an opportunity to enhance and deepen your meditation. We have asked you a few thought-provoking questions to help you get started. Feel free to write or draw. Journal as creatively as you are inspired. This is your time to dream of the supportive connections between your body and nature.

There is much to discover about your relationship with your body and the beautiful world around you. Find a comfortable place to relax and enjoy. Prepare to be transported to a setting where you can unwind, immersed in nature, and experience the unbridled freedom of the wild!

From Wellness To Oneness,

Erik and Faye
Your Virtual Massage Therapists

FROM WELLNESS TO ONENESS

Wherever you are,

however you feel,

whatever your state of wellness,

know that

healing is at hand.

Your body is always seeking balance

and looking for opportunities to restore.

Through wellness,

may you come to oneness

with your body,

your mind,

your spirit,

and the beautiful Earth that supports us all.

ABOUT THIS MEDITATION

Introduction

In wintertime, the vibrant colors of the living world transform into a silvery wonderland. The quietly falling snow brings peace to the wintery world.

Long nights urge us to make the most of the short days.

Snow gives us a chance to explore our world in a completely new way. It makes for a great playground! What great fun it is to ski, snowshoe, sled, and snowboard in the mountains.

Enjoy this story, where you spend a day on a mountain, cross-country skiing to a panoramic vista. See the pristine snow sparkle in the sunlight. Breathe the fresh mountain air. Feel your body warm as your arms and legs move in rhythm.

To glide through the snow in the great outdoors is one of the finest pleasures of winter.

To experience the entire

NatureBody® Connection

scan this QR code

or go to

www.aquaterramassage.com / naturebodygift / winterski

A gift for you, dear reader.

A special reading by the authors awaits you
at the link above.

CHAPTER ONE

The Call of Nature

BREATHING AND GROUNDING

My cozy cabin in the mountains is warm from the heat of the hearth. This cabin is my safe haven, nestled in an evergreen mountain forest.

I look out the window. The snow has fallen gently all night, adding a fresh layer to the winter wonderland. Snow drapes over the tall trees surrounding the cabin. A small bird has left crisp tracks in the white canvas of snow. Winter's cold radiates through the window, contrasting to the comforting warmth within the snug cabin.

My cross-country skis are waiting for me outside, freshly waxed and ready to go. The snow is calling to me. The thoughts of clear sky and crisp air are drawing me outdoors. I will go outside today. I am excited to experience the wonders of winter.

Clothing's Effect on Your Lymphatic System

*"My warm clothes are loose fitting and
I enjoy the freedom of movement they offer."*

From deep tissue massage to light etheric touch, every pressure of massage has different effects on your body. Deep massage influences structures that lie deep within your body: your connective tissue and muscles. Light touch influences the outer layers of your body, like circulation, lymphatic flow, and even the energy emitted outside of your skin.

Our lymphatic system is part of our immune system, transporting white blood cells through our bodies and removing waste. To move lymph during massage, we work at a very light pressure, at the puffy outer layer of your skin. Because the lymph circulates just under your skin, even snug clothing can restrict the flow of lymph. If you notice that you are feeling sore or achy, it could be that your clothing is too tight.

When your low back and hips get achy, notice your waistband. How tight is it? Does it leave an impression on your skin? Is it making you move less freely? Try loosening your belt or switching to loose-fitting clothing.

If your feet are sore, try loosening your shoelaces so your feet can move more freely. Leave room for your toes to wiggle and spread naturally. How tight are your socks? Do they leave imprints on your calves? By dressing in well-fitting clothing, you can help your body move more freely.

I pull on my comfortable wool sweater that keeps me warm even when wet, and an outer jacket for wind and snow. My favorite hat feels soft and comforting as I snuggle it over my ears.

> My warm clothes are loose fitting
> > and I enjoy the freedom of movement they offer.

> I protect myself
> > with a thermal under-layer and a thick outer shell,
> > like a lynx with its densely woven inner fur
> > and longer, courser, outer fur,
> > perfectly designed for winter.

I can wiggle my toes in my flexible cross-country ski boots. My backpack with lunch, water and other necessities completes my outfit.

The Benefits of Nasal Breathing

"I imagine drawing air in through my nose, feeling it warm as it spirals in my sinuses."

Breathing through your nose can have profound health benefits. Your nostrils filter, humidify and warm air before it enters your lungs. Nasal breathing can help you sleep better and has a relaxing effect on your nervous system.[3]

For thousands of years, Indigenous Peoples throughout the Americas warned of the negative health consequences from mouth breathing, cautioning that it led to stress and disease.[4] Nasal breathing was so important to them, they breathed exclusively through their noses, even when running. They trained their children to breathe through their noses from infancy by gently closing their lips after breastfeeding[5] and while they slept.

Nasal breathing changes the chemistry of your breath. When you breathe into your nose, nitric oxide is released into your body. Nitric oxide expands your blood vessels and improves oxygen circulation throughout your body.[6]

Nasal breathing is also relaxing. Breathing deeply through your nose slows your respiration and activates your parasympathetic nervous system, signaling your body to relax.[7]

Nasal breathing can give you an edge on the quality of your respiratory life. Take a breath for strength. Take a breath for stamina. Take a warming, cleansing nasal breath for health.

I head outside. The door creaks as it opens.

The cold, fresh air is invigorating. I quickly close the door behind me to keep the house warm.

I inhale the beautiful crisp evergreen scent of the snowy outside world. The air has drifted down the mountain's steep slopes from glaciers above during the inversion of the night. Filtered through the forest and into my lungs, I relish these refreshing breaths of clean mountain air.

I imagine drawing air in through my nose,
    feeling it warm
    as it spirals in my nostrils.

I picture my breath flowing upward through my sinuses,
    opening the space behind my forehead.

The breath continues,
    curling under my scalp
    and soothing my head.

It flows down the back of my head
    and enters my spine.

My ears relax.

My jaw softens.

The energy of my breath melts down my neck,
    my shoulders,
    my arms,
    and out my hands.

On the Power of Breath

"My next breath comes in through my open sinuses and pours its relaxing energy down my throat, chest, and abdomen."

The breathing meditation in this chapter encourages you to become aware of the sensations of breathing. Visualization can be a powerful tool to breathe deeper and more effectively.

The simple act of breathing is a way for you to invite change into your life. Breathing communicates with all of your body's systems. It coordinates your musculature, your chemistry, and your nervous system.

You can use breathing to influence your physical, mental and energetic self. Breathing can help you relax certain muscles as you stretch or massage them. It can help you strengthen your posture. It can either calm or energize your nervous system. Breathing visualizations can help shape the intentions you have for your body.

Use breath as a creative tool for healing. Breathing can be inspiring in so many ways.

My next breath comes in through my open sinuses
    and pours its relaxing energy down my throat,
    chest,
    and abdomen.

I stretch tall out of my strong legs,
    feeling my hip creases lengthen
    into my long abdomen.

My feet are grounded to the earth
    while my upper body reaches to the sky.

I stand tall,
    and watch,
    and listen.

This peaceful world is silent.

The snow has dampened the sound.

My ears reach and stretch to hear.

My mind is quieted,
    and soothed by silence.

The chilly air exhilarates me. My body is warm and ready to move.

CHAPTER TWO

The Joy of Skiing
BALANCE AND STRENGTH

I drop my skis onto the snow, side by side. Steadying myself with my poles, I step onto each ski, hearing the toes of my flexible ski boots click into place.

I slide my skis back and forth to feel the slipperiness of the snow. The toes of my boots are anchored to my skis, while my heels are free to lift. I am excited for today's ski!

I anchor my poles and strongly slide my lead leg out in front of me, pouring my weight through my foot. I shift my bodyweight to the forward ski, letting my back foot come to toe and lightly glide behind me.

I draw my back leg forward to meet my center.

Developing Powerful Legs

"My powerful thigh muscles become warm as they work."

Your hips and thighs hold some of the most powerful muscles in your body. The strong hamstring and glute muscles in the back of your legs and hips squeeze to propel you forward.

Cross-country skiing simplifies the act of walking, because you do not pick up your feet. Instead of picking up your feet, you slide forward in the tracks. The tracks keep your feet and legs aligned, so your focus can be on opening your front hips and engaging your powerful glutes and hamstrings.

Visualize yourself gliding through the snow. Picture your stride lengthening. Let your front hip open, as the back of your hip and leg fire to you launch into the next step. Imagine your upper body tall and balanced as you strongly slide through the snow.

Whether you are skiing, walking, or running, you can move forward more powerfully by engaging the muscles in the backs of your legs and hips. Enjoy the warmth of firing your muscles as you set your stride for the season.

As my legs zipper back together,
    my weight is evenly balanced on both skis.

My inner thighs work
    to stabilize my centerline.

I slide my other ski forward,
    throwing my weight through my front foot
    to initiate my forward momentum
    and naturally toe with the other foot.

I balance my weight evenly
    to extend my glide.

My pelvis feels level and strong with this motion.

My powerful thigh muscles
    become warm as they work.

My abdomen holds my balance back over my center,
    keeping me from leaning too far forward.

My skis part the pristine, powdery snow,
    creating fresh tracks in its pillowy mounds.

My stride is long and elegant.

A rush of pleasure fills me
    as I think less about the mechanics of the motion
    and focus on the joy of gliding smoothly
    over the soft snow.

Walking to Think Clearly

*"The spiraling energy travels through my body,
two hemispheres working in conjunction."*

One of the best ways to develop our brains began as infants. We had to crawl before we learned to walk. Crawling created connections between the two halves of our brain.[8] The integration of the two hemispheres unleashed our ability to focus and learn more easily. As adults, walking continues to coordinate our ability to concentrate and think clearly.

Each hemisphere of the brain controls movement on the opposite side of the body.[9] In order to crawl, walk, run, ski, or swim, one leg moves forward while the opposite arm swings. This full-body, rhythmic movement helps to build the bridge between the two hemispheres of our brain. Electrical impulses pass more freely between the left and right brain, improving our energy and focus.[10]

Each side of your brain plays its own role in helping you with any activity you do, whether you are writing, playing an instrument or a sport, or even juggling. It is important that the right and left brain work together, to learn intricate skills and help you achieve more complex goals.[11]

When you need to focus your mind and balance your energy, try your favorite cross-lateral activity. Walking is one of the simplest cross-lateral activities. Every step strengthens your ability to take the next: physically and neurologically. Walk to free your mind and feel your body thrive!

As my body warms,
*   my stride lengthens.*

My front hips open long and wide
*   while my hamstrings and glutes launch me stronger*
*   into the next step.*

I ski toward two parallel depressions in the snow. Yesterday's
ski tracks have been covered by the fresh flakes of last night.
As I drop into the tracks, I feel the solid packed snow under
my skis: smooth, satin ribbons in the snow.

The movement of my skis in snow feels silky.
*   They skim lightly along the tracks.*

My body relaxes into a moving meditation.

I pole in opposite time to my skis,
*   allowing my sides and abs*
*   to help counterbalance*
*   the strong motion of my legs.*

My poles work to keep me centered over my skis.

Acting like the ama of an outrigger canoe,
*   a pole helps me stabilize*
*   as I balance all the weight on one foot,*
*   and then shift to the other.*

One arm reaches forward with the opposite leg.

The spiraling energy travels through my body,
*   two hemispheres working in conjunction.*

Leg Springs

"The effort of my leg muscles spirals around bone like great coils of energy."

Your leg muscles are some of the most powerful muscles of your body. They are meant to support and balance you, protect your joints, and propel you across the earth. To walk smoothly, muscles, tendons and ligaments coordinate to bend and straighten your legs like dynamic coils.

Cats fluidly coordinate their movements to walk silently and smoothly. Visualize moving with the finesse of a cat, prowling and padding quietly. With your hips, knees and ankles slightly bent, feel your feet conforming to the ground under you. Let your toes be soft as you finish your step. Your leg muscles are becoming supple and efficient.

Imagine you are using your legs like springs. Your leg muscles wrap around the bones, like great, powerful coils. Your knees, hips, and ankles load and release as you move.

The more your leg muscles fire, the stronger they become. They carry your body more easily and help you to stand up taller. Strong legs keep you balanced and springing gracefully across the earth.

My sternum and hips stay square to the path.

I engage my abs to lengthen my spine
    and float my upper body through the glide.

I am skiing! Glistening crystals of snow sparkle in the sun's
rays before me.

Fresh air intoxicates me with spirit.
    It cools my brain as it slips into my nose
    and passes over the roof of my mouth and throat.

I relish the contrast of the cool air in my warm body,
    smooth and flowing.

My powerful legs continue to work
    and propel me forward along the path.

The effort of my leg muscles spirals around bone
    like great coils of energy.

I load and release this energy
    using my legs like springs.

My skis slide softly over this frozen world.

The Weightlessness of Strength

"The more I bend my knees, allowing my powerful legs to be explosive in their effort, the more I feel weightless..."

Visualizing and working toward stronger muscles gives us the freedom to move more effortlessly. We gain more control over our bodies and become more graceful.

Bending and flexing our knees can build powerful leg muscles that are ready to help us move in any direction. Our leg muscles cushion and protect our bodies from the impact of walking and movement. Strong leg muscles help us become more nimble.

With every step you take, your body gets a little stronger. Every time you stretch, your muscles become a little longer. Breathing gives your muscles the oxygen they need to relax more completely and contract more powerfully. With each glass of water you drink, your body becomes more fluid and supple.

As your muscles become stronger, you overcome gravity more easily. You are able to move more freely. A strong, graceful stride can make you feel like you are floating across the floor.

Have faith that change can happen. Let your malleable muscles be your inspiration for change, growth and healing.

The trail follows a little creek for a while. Icy water babbles between the snowy banks. Exposed river stones are covered by soft, rounded clumps of snow.

A small winter bird alights on a snow-covered rock in the brook. It peers into the icy water, and then disappears, submerging its plumply feathered body completely. It pops back up onto the ice-rimmed rocks again with an impressively earned meal: a tiny bug from the aquatic world.

I find my stride again on the silky path.

> *The rhythm of skiing takes over*
> *and I feel graceful as I glide smoothly.*

> *The more I bend my knees,*
> *allowing my powerful legs to be explosive in their effort,*
> *the more I feel weightless,*
> *like I am floating over the snow.*

> *I listen to the swish of my skis.*

CHAPTER THREE

Breathing With the Mountain

PULMONARY OPENING,
HIP AND SHOULDER MASSAGE

Evergreen trees rise out of the snow on either side of the path. They are sleeping in this frozen world. Their cold sap slows as they wait out the winter months, patiently growing the fresh buds of spring.

Small birds dart around snowy branches. These little gray jays are friendly and fearless and watch me closely to see if there will be any opportunities for snacks. The bravest birds dart lower in the trees, perching in nearby branches. They cock their heads to the side as they watch me.

There is an incline ahead. Snow sparkles between the crisp shadows of snow-flocked trees, painting the trail in black and white.

I launch myself uphill, pulling my knees up powerfully as the back of my legs stretch long.

The Flow of Exercise

"My muscles, heart, and breath work as one."

During our long days of trekking on the Appalachian Trail, we came to understand a few things about how the body reaches its daily performance level.

With any exercise, it takes time for your muscles and breathing to "warm up." As you warm up, your body can feel tired and sore for the first twenty minutes or so. Your breathing can feel labored and uncomfortable.

This soon changes as your body finds its rhythm.

The next forty minutes can have a range of feelings while your body adjusts. When you start to get into the flow of the activity, your body moves better. Your breathing finds a rhythm in harmony with your movement. Your endorphins kick in and soreness subsides. Your mind clears with each exhale. You feel great. You start experiencing the sought-after "runner's high."

Time slips by. You are present in the moment.

Your motions take less concentration. You begin to be more aware of what is around you. Exercise becomes a moving meditation.

Endure the time of warming up to enjoy the rhythm of moving. Movement supports the flow of your life.

As I ascend,
  my heart beats strongly.
  I breathe vigorously.

I am present in the moment
  as I focus on my stride.

My muscles, heart, and breath work as one.

I feel the rhythm of my breath
  and the drumming of my heart
  in the performance of my muscles.

In a particularly steep section of trail, I angle my skis into a
v-shape. I dig the inside edge of my skis into the snow. Step
by step, this herringbone pattern of skiing gets me up the
hill.

My strong glutes and thighs are fully activated.

My inner leg leads my steps
  in this out-turned stance.

When one leg begins to slip,
  I widen the V-shape of my stance even farther.

I press strongly into my poles
  to balance the effort.

The motion of my arms
  brings length to my spine.
  The crown of my head reaches up
  out of my long neck.

Loping Like a Wolf

"My breathing eases to a comfortable rhythm in my natural, loping pace."

Wolves cover great distances using a trotting lope, conserving energy with their efficient stride. They can keep this pace for hours, sometimes traveling sixty miles in a night.

A wolf's stride is easy, springy, and long. When it lifts its paw, its ankle is loose and relaxed. The wolf keeps its muscles relaxed until it needs them. Then it contracts its muscles strongly and explosively. This focused use of its muscles gives the wolf an efficient stride that allows it to cover great distances.

We can learn a lot from the way wolves lope. If we keep our muscles loose and relaxed, we can maximize our strength and efficiency, and enjoy the fun of exercise. Sore muscles are tight muscles. A tight muscle is "on." It is already working. A relaxed muscle, on the other hand, has all of its fibers available to use. Being able to let your muscles relax between contractions makes you stronger and able to go farther, like the wolf.

Notice your stride. Are there moments when your muscles feel soft and loose? Stretch and massage your muscles. Shake off the tension by literally shaking your limbs and bouncing around. Let your muscles flop around like water balloons. As your muscles release unnecessary holding, they become more available for play.

When the slope eases, I return my skis to the tracks and press forward in my familiar glide. Progress quickens on this easier slope and my muscles clear the soreness of the climb.

My breathing eases to a comfortable rhythm
in my natural, loping pace.

I work to be strong enough
to maintain my glide uphill,
balancing my weight across the faces of both skis.

I throw my weight forward onto my front ski,
carrying my force forward.

As I glide,
I keep weight in my back ski
to help me stay balanced.

I crest the hill and see the view open before me: a brilliant crystalline world under a deep blue sky.

CHAPTER FOUR

Stillness in the Flow

A FULL BODY RELAXATION

I coast peacefully along the ridge. My breathing is steady. My legs and arms move together in smooth rhythm.

After a long climb and a short run along the ridge, I reach the top of the hill. I look back down the mountain. My two tracks, leading between the trees, disappear into the forest.

A view of the valley spills out before me, lined by distant, snow-capped mountains. Nestled in the heart of this valley is a frozen mountain lake. My cozy cabin awaits on its shore.

Up here, the sky is a deep shade of blue. It is as if I am closer to the edge of the atmosphere. The deep blue sky intensifies the brilliance of the white snow.

The Weight of Relaxation

"I let my body become heavier."

There are times when it is difficult to relax. The more we try to "make" ourselves relax, the more tense we seem to become. Trying to relax can be stressful!

One way to bring your body into relaxation is to approach relaxation a little differently. Instead of trying to surrender into relaxation, you can proactively focus on breathing to relax. Inhale as if you were breathing into the tension. Fill it with air. Feel yourself become heavier as you exhale. Let the tension float away. This technique works well for your whole body, or a specific area.

Let us use our shoulders as an example. Begin by noticing the tension in your shoulders. Where do you feel the tightest? Expand those tight tissues with your inhale. On your next exhale, let your shoulders become heavier. You can accentuate this release by gently pulling your shoulders downward to strengthen the opposing muscles.

Breathe. Feel your muscles become a little heavier on each exhale.

Be patient. It can take several repetitions to let the tension go.

Enjoy the feeling of your body sinking into relaxation.

I find a nice sunny spot out of the breeze to rest. I remove my pack and sitting pad. I towel off my moist skin, and put on my hat and gloves to retain the warmth I have earned. Refreshed and toasty, I recline back on the insulated pad in the snow.

My body forms into the fluffy snow, which yields to create the perfect depression for my body, like nature's beanbag.

I am perfectly warm in the winter sunshine.

I breathe gently,
> *and let the breath flow down into my low belly*
> *as my muscles relax.*
> *My belly softens.*

My legs feel warm and energized
> *from the workout.*

My breathing slows
> *and my back stretches across the snow.*

I let my body become heavier.

The silence of the forest, shrouded in snow,
> *drops down over my ears.*

I listen deeply to the quiet around me.

The muted world
> *carries serenity in its silence,*
> *like a blanket over me.*

On Moving Freely

"I imagine what it must feel like to run freely across the powdery snowfields without sinking."

How can I move with the fluid effortlessness of a loping wolf? Freedom in our bodies begins with an idea: a vision that our bodies can mimic and strive toward.

Picture the wolf. Imagine it gliding smoothly forward. Notice its legs stretching into a long stride... its head and neck relaxed as it casually glances around... its strong core supporting its movement.

As you imagine moving like the wolf, begin with your center. When your abdominal muscles engage, they support your center of gravity. They contain your middle so your limbs can move strong and free. Your strong legs propel you forward. Your shoulders and arms swing to help you increase your speed and steady your balance. Your neck and head are free to swivel and take in the world around you. You begin to move more effortlessly.

By imagining these nuances of feeling, even if it just seems like a dreamy fantasy, you give your amazing mind and talented body the opportunity to step in and perform together in ways that we cannot consciously understand. Your visualization of the wolf composes a symphony of movement. These thoughts unleash your body to perform and to function. You achieve a feeling from an idea that you perceived in a moment of clarity.

My brain releases its effort toward trying to hear
and enjoys the purity of this silent, snowy world.

The sun feels refreshing.
I close my eyes and angle my face toward its warmth.

My calm breathing is rhythmic and measured.

I allow the sun's warmth to sink through my body,
calming me into a peaceful state.

I take in the world around me. I notice the tracks of a rabbit in the snow. It traveled close to the brush that keeps it hidden and provides forage through the lean winter months.

As my eyes take in more detail, smaller tracks come into focus. The small feet of a tiny mouse have left delicate patterns in the snow. It barely made an imprint with its lightweight body. I imagine what it must feel like to run freely across the powdery snowfields without sinking.

The sun's heat warms the snow in the trees. A heavily weighted branch releases a clump of snow, striking the ground with a soft thump.

I am blissfully present
in this silent place on top of the world.

Your Atmosphere

*"The atmosphere itself, the precious, thin, silken veil
over our whole planet, gives me the sense that
I am sitting in the most picturesque scene of a snow globe."*

Our atmosphere provides protection, making our planet a habitable, welcoming home for life. It deflects harmful radiation and provides friction to burn up meteorites. Oxygen, moisture, and mild temperatures abound in Earth's protective atmosphere.

As you build a kinder, more compassionate relationship with your body, you are creating your own protective atmosphere. You get to decide what you leave out, and what you allow in. What types of activity, food, thought, and relationships do you want to invite into your life? Which of these no longer have a place in your protected inner atmosphere?

Building a healthy relationship with your body allows you to be malleable and resilient with the outside world, while you thrive and feel safe within.

May the life you visualize in your snow globe be full, rich and beautiful.

The heavy flowing effort to arrive here has been replaced by the stillness of being here. With my mind and body at rest, my spirit longs to see the connections in the world around me.

The snow upon which I sit
may one day fill the lake in the valley below.

The oxygen of the trees
will one day fill the great blue sky.

The atmosphere itself, the precious, thin, silken veil over our whole planet, gives me the sense that I am sitting in the most picturesque scene of a snow globe.

CHAPTER FIVE

Down to the Lake

LOWER BODY MASSAGE

After a refreshing rest, I pack up and clip on my skis. This will be a fun downhill glide. I will enjoy the silky texture and extra speed of my freshly laid tracks.

The hill slopes gently down ahead of me. I open my stride and begin to descend. My skis effortlessly slide through the tracks.

I direct my movement with my core.

> *My inner thighs engage*
> *to keep my feet magnetized together in the tracks.*

> *I keep my knees slightly bent,*
> *and move from my center,*
> *just below my belly button.*

The Adaptable Body

---

*"I lengthen my stride with strong glutes,
opening my front hip flexors."*

Our bodies adapt to every activity we do. If we sit for extended periods, our hips respond by shortening in the front and stretching in the back. When we stand up again, our shortened front hips can tilt our pelvis forward. This change in balance and muscle tone can lead to a sore back.

You can remind your body of its natural posture by stretching the front of your legs and hips, and strengthening your glute muscles. Walking, running and skiing are great exercises to help activate your glute muscles. As you strengthen and stretch your hips, your pelvis becomes rebalanced and the extra pressure is taken off your low back.

Better posture can help you become more effective at your work, your activities, and your hobbies. When you work on your posture, your muscles respond. Your body is great at adapting to what you ask of it.

Cool air drifts past my face as I glide downhill. I kick once in a while to keep my speed up. I have found my rhythm.

I lengthen my stride with strong glutes,
    opening my front hip flexors.

My body feels more graceful
    as I rise up out of my core.

My legs feel longer and lighter.

My arms swing effortlessly
    as they support my balanced progress.

I am relaxing through the movement.

My skis and poles are becoming more of an extension of me.

As my skis slide over small rises in the trail,
    I stay centered over my feet and allow my knees to bend,
    keeping my body spring-like.

I kick off the back of these mounds
    to keep up my speed.

At the bottom of the hill, the trail flattens and I resume my familiar, loping stride. I feel warm. My motion is smooth.

Rather than going directly back to the cabin, I take the long way home along the shores of the mountain lake.

The lake is frozen and blanketed in snow. I ski along the treelined shore, looking out at the white openness.

A Season for Rest

"Life has slowed for the season."

Winter is a time for rest.

After the renewal of spring, the expansive growth of summer, and the autumn harvest, winter is the season of returning to center.

From the push of growth to the drawing back toward dormancy, our world, and our bodies, have a natural rhythm. We need both actions to be healthy.

Allow yourself to rest. Give yourself the time to sleep and dream. Welcome periods of inactivity, of daydreaming, and imagination, into your life. They can be real sources of inspiration.

There is so much more to you than what you achieve. You are greater than a human "doing." Allow yourself to experience "being."

In the summertime, wildlife will return to the high mountain slopes, and find nourishment and refuge near the shores of this lake. It will be full of activity. Water bugs will hover above the lake in the warm summer light. Lily pads will grace the shallows. The summertime world will be abuzz in sound and aflame in color.

But now, there is a hushed quiet as soft snow covers the terrain. Life has slowed for the season. Small mammals are tucked away in cozy burrows, keeping each other warm by snuggling close. Fish have drifted deeper down in the cold, viscous water. I imagine them slowly curving their silvery bodies back and forth among the grasses at the bottom of the frigid lake.

The forest floor is deeply covered by snow. In peaceful dormancy, plant life has slowed its growth for the season. Spring bulbs patiently wait for their chance to unfurl and flourish. The world is fast asleep in its seasonal slumber.

The blanket of snow dampens sound.

A quiet hush resonates across the landscape.

This is the time for peace.
    For reflection.
    For meditation.

My body feels warm and glowing.

As the sunlight fades, the cool of the evening presses through my clothes. In the distance I see my cozy cabin, the warm glow from its windows casting an amber light on the blue evening snow. I ski back toward its comforting warmth and the promise of a relaxing evening by the fire.

CHAPTER SIX

Gratitude

A BLESSING FROM THE WINTER

T hank you for joining me on this adventure. Together, we have witnessed the quiet strength of the mountain on this winter day. Until we meet again,

May your heart be a source of warmth
for all those who seek its coziness.

May your mind feel as free
as the vista from the mountaintops.

May your circulation flow
as smoothly as skis on snow.

May your muscles spring and contract
in anticipation of the seasons to come.

On Gratitude

"Together, we have witnessed the quiet strength
of the mountain on this winter day."

Thank you.

The simplest prayer.

It is a wonder that some of the simplest things in life can be so profoundly beneficial. Giving thanks has been shown to have positive effects on our health. Gratitude can reduce stress hormones, decrease blood pressure, and improve heart rate variability.[12] It improves our outlook and the quality of our sleep.[13]

Try giving thanks daily.

Notice how your perspective changes.

May you tap into the patient, peaceful stillness
in your own being.

May the rhythm of your heart and breath
strongly support the dreams of your soul.

And when it is time to light your fire,
be sure to open your flue and breathe.

Glide on, Tranquil Wanderer.

Acknowledgments

Some of my favorite memories growing up were the winter days I spent cross country skiing with my parents, Bonny and David Erickson. Thank you for introducing me to the mountains.

James Nestor's book, Breathing: The New Science of A Lost Art, is a fascinating and engaging read that discusses how the simple act of breathing can help or harm your health.

We have enjoyed NOAA's interesting infographics on weather patterns. Thank you for sharing the information.

I am grateful to Donna Eden, author of the book, *Energy Medicine,* for showing me how energy can affect your body. I attended a workshop with her many years ago that still returns to my mind occasionally. Her enlightening talk on the cross-crawl pattern inspired me to think more about how moving our bodies can affect how we think.

Since I was little, I have felt inspired by the last line of the Little Golden Book, Heidi, adapted from the book by Johanna Spyri. After a healing summer in the Alps, Heidi's friend, Clara, recovered from a long illness. Heidi danced around Clara, singing, "I knew the mountains would make you well! I knew they would make you well!"

May the mountains heal us all.

Notes

1. "What is Imagery?" *Johns Hopkins Medicine,* 2003, www.hopkinsmedicine.org/health/wellness-and-prevention/imagery.

2. Lohr, Jim. "Can Visualizing Your Body Doing Something Help You Learn to Do It Better?" *Scientific American,* 1 May 2015, www.scientificamerican.com/article/can-visualizing-your-body-doing-something-help-you-learn-to-do-it-better.

3. Gross, Terry. "How The 'Lost Art' Of Breathing Can Impact Sleep And Resilience." *National Public Radio,* 27 May 2020, www.npr.org/sections/health-shots/2020/05/27/862963172/how-the-lost-art-of-breathing-can-impact-sleep-and-resilience.

4. Nestor, James. "Why Nasal Breathing Matters, Now More Than Ever." *MindBodyGreen,* 2 June 2020, www.mindbodygreen.com/articles/health-benefits-of-breathing-through-your-nose.

5. Nestor, James. "Part Two-The Lost Art and Science of Breathing." *Breath: The New Science of A Lost Art,* Riverhead Books, 2020, pp. 46-49.

6. Malaguti, Luca. "Breathe Through Your Nose! The Science of Breathing & Nasal Nitric Oxide." *Freedive Wire,* 15 September 2022, www.freedivewire.com/science-breathing-nasal-nitric-oxide.

7. Panasevich, Jake. "Nasal Breathing: the Secret to Optimal Fitness?" *US News and World Report,* 7 September 2020, health.usnews.com/health-news/blogs/eat-run/articles/nasal-breathing-the-secret-to-optimal-fitness.

8. Horner, Cynthia. "The Importance of Crawling for an Infant" *Dr. Cynthia Horner-Chiropractor,* 13 August 2014, www.drcynthiahorner.com/crawling-important-for-an-infant.

9. "Brain." *Cleveland Clinic,* 30 March 2022, my.clevelandclinic.org/health/body/22638-brain.

10. Curtain, Melanie. "Want to Sync the 2 Hemispheres of Your Brain? Neuroscience Says to Do This Daily. (It Only Takes 4 Minutes)." *Inc,* 29 December 2019, www.inc.com/melanie-curtin/want-to-sync-2-hemispheres-of-your-brain-neuroscience-says-to-do-this-daily-it-only-takes-4-minutes.html.

11. Kabel, Olga. "How to integrate your right and left brain through movement." *SequenceWiz,* 13 August 2014, sequencewiz.org/2014/08/13/integrating-right-and-left-brain.

12. McCraty, R., Barrios-Choplin, B., Rozman, D., Atkinson, M., & Watkins, A. D. "The impact of a new emotional self-management program on stress, emotions, heart rate variability, DHEA and cortisol." *Integrative Physiological and Behavioral Science: The Official Journal of the Pavlovian Society,* vol 33, no. 2, 1998, pp. 151–170, doi.org/10.1007/BF02688660.

13. Digdon, N., & Koble, A. "Effects of Constructive Worry, Imagery Distraction, and Gratitude Interventions on Sleep Quality: A Pilot Trial." *Applied Psychology: Health and Well-being,* vol. 3, no. 2, 2011, pp. 193-206, doi.org/10.1111/j.1758-0854.2011.01049.x.

MEDITATION

Journal

This journal gives you a place to reflect on your experience as you read and meditate. With every meditation, your library of personal affirmations can grow. Some thoughts you might want to record, in words or drawings, are:

What were your favorite phrases or ideas in the story?

Did you find yourself standing taller as you contemplated your long hip flexors and strong glute muscles? How did it feel?

Talk about stillness. How do you give yourself time to rest?

Make a list of the things for which you are grateful. What sensations do you notice in your body as you focus on gratitude?

How can you make more space for mindfulness in your life? Are there ways for you to feel less busy, so you have more time to be? What part of your life needs your mindful time now?

"I RELISH THESE REFRESHING BREATHS OF CLEAN MOUNTAIN AIR."

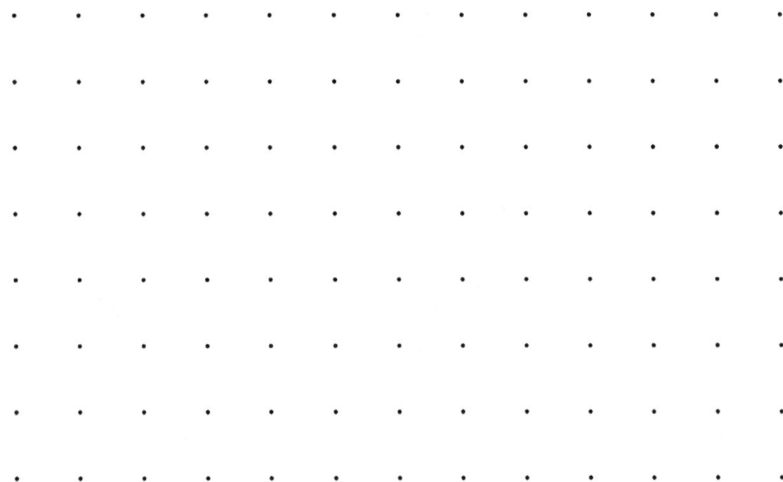

MEDITATION

When you open a window and enjoy a fresh breeze, you are letting in air that has traveled all around the world. It has drifted over snowy mountains, traveled through serene valleys, gusted across wild oceans, and floated into your window. Now it is here for you.

Exhale this air back into the world, and set it free to continue its journey around this beautiful planet.

You are connected to all that is.

~

May your

HEART

be a source of warmth

for all those

who seek its coziness.

May your

MIND

feel as free

as the vista

from the mountaintops.

"I AM PURELY IN THE MOMENT
AS I FOCUS ON MY STRIDE."

MEDITATION

There is a special time when your body is warmed up and you are focused on what you are doing. Being present while you move through your day is a form of moving meditation. It is a feeling of being "in the flow."

~

May your

CIRCULATION

flow as smoothly

as skis on snow.

> "THE WORLD IS FAST ASLEEP IN ITS SEASONAL SLUMBER."

MEDITATION

Winter is the season of slumber. Animals and insects have made their winter homes underground, and are quietly resting until spring. The plant world is dormant, waiting for spring to send new shoots upwards. Even daylight has quieted, fading into long, starlit nights.

Honor your body in this dreamy, dark season. Take time to renew and be at peace. You are resting alongside the slumbering life on this planet, connected in dreams.

~

May your

MUSCLES

spring and contract

in anticipation

of the seasons to come.

"THE SILENCE OF THE SNOWY DAY DROPS OVER MY EARS. I LISTEN DEEPLY TO THE QUIET AROUND ME."

MEDITATION

L isten to the sounds around you. Now listen deeper. Underneath sound, there is a quiet stillness. Bring your awareness to that silent place. How do you feel? What thoughts come to you as you focus on stillness?

~

May you

tap into the

patient,

PEACEFUL

STILLNESS

in your own being.

"SNOW DRAPES OVER THE TALL
TREES."

MEDITATION

I magine yourself a tree in winter. Snow gently covers you like a blanket. Its comforting presence weights your shoulders and drifts down your arms. Feel your jaw softening, your chest relaxing, and your breathing calming. Let your neck lengthen as your crown rises up toward the sky. Feel balance return to your body.

~

May the

rhythm of your

HEART

and

BREATH

support the dreams

of your soul.

When it is time to

LIGHT

YOUR

FIRE

be sure to open

your flue and breathe.

"GLISTENING CRYSTALS OF SNOW
SPARKLE IN THE SUN'S RAYS
BEFORE ME."

MEDITATION

B eauty exists everywhere. From the panoramic magnificence of a towering mountain range, to the tiniest flake of snow, glinting as it refract the sun's rays, magic and beauty are all around you.

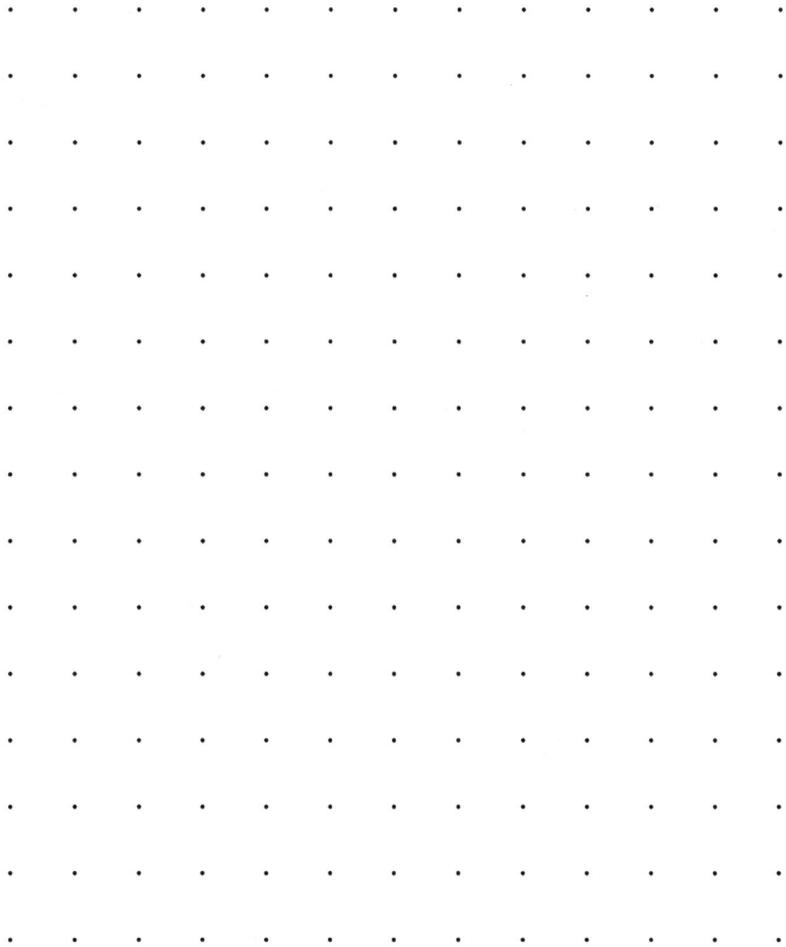

~

BLESSING
FROM THE WINTER

May your
HEART
be a source of warmth
for all those who seek its coziness.

May your
MIND
feel as free
as the vista from the mountaintops.

May your
CIRCULATION
flow as smoothly as skis on snow.

May your
MUSCLES
spring and contract
in anticipation of the seasons to come.

May you tap into the patient, peaceful
STILLNESS
in your own being.

May the rhythm of your
HEART AND BREATH
strongly support the dreams of your soul.

And when it is time to
LIGHT YOUR FIRE
be sure to open your flue and breathe.

About the Authors

Born and raised in New Orleans, Erik Krippner grew up with a po'boy in his hand and a song in his heart. As a boy, he spent his summers swimming, hiking, fishing, and sailing. After becoming an Eagle Scout, Erik dreamed of answering the call to "Go West, young man." He earned a Bachelor of Science degree in Forestry from Louisiana State University. Following his passion for adventure, Erik found his way to the mountains of the Pacific Northwest, his home to this day. After working in the forests of Oregon, Washington, Idaho, Alaska, Georgia, and Louisiana, Erik decided to focus his love of natural sciences on the study of human body through massage therapy.

Faye grew up in Oregon surrounded by family and old growth coastal forests. She spent many childhood weekends cross-country skiing, hunting for mushrooms, exploring coastal tide pools, and searching for crawdads in the Siuslaw River. Her love of books deepened when she became the editor of her high school and college's literary journals. Upon earning her Bachelor of Arts degree in Mathematics with honors from the Robert D. Clark Honors College at the University of Oregon, Faye became a technical writer and web developer. The whisper of a deeper purpose ignited her to study massage, where she met Erik.

Erik and Faye became friends in massage school at the East West College of the Healing Arts, in Portland, Oregon. In 2003, they founded Aqua Terra Massage, a therapeutic massage studio for friends and couples. Since then, they have practiced therapeutic massage together, side by side. They have spent years immersed in the study of massage, serving thousands of clients.

Faye and Erik have spent years exploring and writing about our beautiful world. They have sailed the blue waters of Fiji's Koro Sea, kayaked New Zealand's Marlborough Sound, and stargazed among the giraffes and elephants in Botswana. They have hiked the Appalachian Trail and paddled the tidally-influenced Columbia River in the Pacific Northwest. They have seen orca whales swim right under their kayaks, locked eyes with wild lions, and played hide-and-seek with an octopus. They have hiked thousands of miles together, kayaked and sailed hundreds, and spent countless evenings camping under the stars.

With a commitment to bringing more love and kindness
to this beautiful world, we offer this book to you.

www.aquaterramassage.com

www.ingramcontent.com/pod-product-compliance
Lightning Source LLC
Chambersburg PA
CBHW071404050426

42335CB00063B/1627